ALEJANDRO VILLAO RODRÍGUEZ
SILVIA LARA ARRIAGA

The pedagogical role of the teaching physician

ALEJANDRO VILLAO RODRÍGUEZ
SILVIA LARA ARRIAGA

The pedagogical role of the teaching physician

in the training of medical students in obstetrical emergency care

ScienciaScripts

Imprint

Any brand names and product names mentioned in this book are subject to trademark, brand or patent protection and are trademarks or registered trademarks of their respective holders. The use of brand names, product names, common names, trade names, product descriptions etc. even without a particular marking in this work is in no way to be construed to mean that such names may be regarded as unrestricted in respect of trademark and brand protection legislation and could thus be used by anyone.

Cover image: www.ingimage.com

This book is a translation from the original published under ISBN 978-613-9-40610-4.

Publisher:
Sciencia Scripts
is a trademark of
Dodo Books Indian Ocean Ltd. and OmniScriptum S.R.L publishing group

120 High Road, East Finchley, London, N2 9ED, United Kingdom
Str. Armeneasca 28/1, office 1, Chisinau MD-2012, Republic of Moldova, Europe
Printed at: see last page
ISBN: 978-620-7-90409-9

"THE PEDAGOGICAL ROLE OF THE TEACHING PHYSICIAN IN THE TRAINING OF MEDICAL STUDENTS FOR OBSTETRIC EMERGENCY CARE."

ALEJANDRO VILLAO RODRIGUEZ

alejandro_villao@hotmail.com
Independent researcher *Orcid 0009-0003-9132-9206 Guayaquil - Ecuador*

SILVIA LARA ARRIAGA

silviamlaraa@hotmail.com
Independent Researcher
*Orcid: 0000-0002-0964-6751
Guayaquil - Ecuador*

Correspondence Author: Alejandro Villao Rodríguez

+593 991912092

Alejandro_villao@hotmail.com

Conflicts of Interest: None to declare.

SUMMARY

In this article, an exhaustive exploration of the pedagogical role of the teaching physician in the training of medical students in obstetric emergency care was carried out. The research, based on interviews with teaching physicians specializing in this field, revealed a central thesis that highlights the crucial importance of the teaching physician as a guide, leader, and ethical role model in the training process. In response to common challenges, such as variability in clinical experience and time management, adaptive and flexible approaches were identified as effective strategies. Adaptation emerged as a key element to personalize teaching, incorporating realistic simulations, problem-based learning and educational technologies. While the promotion of active participation and hands-on learning, through interactive scenarios and discussions based on real cases, was established as essential in the educational process. The inclusion of ethics and cultural sensitivity in teaching was recognized as a key factor in training culturally competent medical professionals. Also, educational technologies, such as advanced simulators and virtual reality, were highlighted as effective tools to improve training in obstetric emergencies. The unified conclusion of the article emphasized the urgent need for continuing education for teaching physicians, with participation in scientific events and collaboration with experts as essential strategies. In summary, the retrospective analysis presented in this article reveals a holistic and adaptive approach to teaching obstetric emergencies, outlining effective practices that have left a positive imprint on the training of future medical professionals.

Key words:

Obstetric emergencies, teaching physician, adaptive teaching, educational technologies, continuing education.

INTRODUCTION

The training of medical students is an intricate process that encompasses not only the transmission of knowledge, but also the cultivation of practical skills and ethical values. In the health care setting, training in obstetric emergencies takes on a singular importance due to the critical nature of these situations for maternal and fetal health. Within such contextualization, the teaching physician emerges as a key figure, playing a fundamental role in the guidance and training of future medical professionals (1).

When entering emergency obstetric care, medical students face a complex terrain that demands not only acute technical skills, but also the ability to make quick and ethical decisions under pressure. Training should be designed in a comprehensive manner, simulating realistic scenarios that allow students to develop both technical skills and the empathy necessary to address the emotional and ethical complexities of emergency obstetrics.

The teaching physician assumes the crucial role of facilitator and guide in this educational process, since beyond being a mere transmitter of information, the teaching physician creates an educational environment that encourages active participation, problem solving and the development of interpersonal skills. This is because their pedagogical role involves not only teaching theoretical knowledge, but also modeling behaviors and attitudes that students should incorporate into their professional practice (2).

The relationship between the teaching physician and the students is fundamental for the integral formation, whose teaching of obstetric emergencies is not only about the acquisition of technical skills, but also about the intemalization of ethical values. In which the teaching physician transmits the importance of empathy, effective communication and respect towards patients in critical situations, thus contributing to the humanization of medical care.

In the training process, the teaching physician not only instructs on procedures and protocols, but also encourages reflection and self-evaluation. In which ethical decision making and the ability to handle delicate situations become fundamental skills that are cultivated throughout the training. Within which the teacher acts as a mentor, guiding students towards a deep understanding of the ethical and emotional responsibilities involved in obstetric emergency care (3).

Obstetric emergency care demands not only technical competence, but also a special sensitivity to the emotional needs of patients. In this sense, the teaching physician, through his interaction with students, models patient-centered care, where the humanization of medicine becomes a fundamental principle.

It should be emphasized that the teaching physician, by assuming his pedagogical role, contributes to the formation of medical professionals who are not only technically competent, but also ethically and humanistically competent. Whose teaching of obstetric emergencies becomes an integral process, where the teaching physician, as a guide, molds not only the students' clinical skills, but also their capacity to face ethical challenges with compassion and judgment (4).

Therefore, training medical students in obstetric emergencies is not only about transmitting knowledge and practical skills, but also about establishing a meaningful connection between the teaching physician and the trainees. Where the mentoring relationship becomes a crucial element for the success of the training, as it allows for a more effective transfer of knowledge and experience. The teaching physician, by building a strong bond with the trainees, facilitates a learning environment in which trust and open communication are essential.

Similarly, it is essential to emphasize that the teaching physician is not only limited to teaching in the academic setting, but also plays an active role in introducing students to real clinical situations. Since early exposure to practical cases under the direct supervision of the teaching physician allows students to apply their theoretical knowledge in a practical setting. Such early immersion contributes to the development of the confidence and competence necessary to address future obstetric emergencies independently (5).

The diversity of clinical scenarios in obstetric emergencies presents an additional challenge in training, in which the teaching physician, by exposing students to a variety of cases, ensures that they are prepared to face the complexity and unpredictability that characterize this area of medicine. Where comprehensive training includes not only common situations, but also those that present unique challenges, thus fostering adaptability and resilience in students.

Based on the above, it can be inferred that the pedagogical role of the teaching physician in the training of medical students for obstetric emergency care is essential for the development of well-rounded and ethical health professionals. Through guidance, supervision and behavioral modeling, the teaching physician plays a crucial role in the training of future experts in obstetric emergency care, preparing them to address not only the technical complexities, but also the ethical and emotional aspects of this critical area of medicine.

METHODOLOGY

Basic research modality

This research is defined as a methodical, systematic, objective and structured process that aims to answer a series of questions, theories, hypotheses and assumptions that arise on a given topic "The pedagogical role of the teaching physician in the training of medical students for obstetric emergency care". The main objective of this study is to investigate the impact of the pedagogical role of the teaching physician in the training of medical students for the care of obstetric emergencies, for which it is important to generate knowledge, changing ideas, providing instant solutions to everyday problems from the observations of the researcher.

Descriptive research

The descriptive research has the task of determining the characteristics of the target population, its methodology is focused on answering the question of the legal problem, it also aims to describe the nature of the demographic segments rather than the causes of the phenomenon, all this through the use of an autonomous didactic matrix based on the psychological damage caused by informal work.

Bibliographic research

Bibliographic research can be defined as any work that requires gathering information from websites that are used to obtain accurate information. These can include more traditional sources such as books, magazines, newspapers and reviews, as well as electronic media such as audio and video recordings and films, and online sources such as websites, which are the most popular sources for confirming prior knowledge.

Field research

All field research is based on conducting a series of observations, interviews and analysis of the people involved. Large companies may have their own marketing or research departments that collect data from primary sources. For this reason, most fieldwork focuses on external organizations that conduct surveys, focus groups and interviews on behalf of the company. Field research work is the collection of new data from primary sources for a specific purpose. This can also be taken as a qualitative data collection method to understand, observe and interact with people in a given socio-cultural context.

Methods used in this study

Qualitative method:

The qualitative method is an analytical tool designed mainly for problem solvers to understand the psyche behind each problem (observe, listen and understand), this requires a rigorous systematization of the various methods and tools that make up the methodological acquis and, therefore, an excellent knowledge of the theory, the implementation of this method is essential because it will allow us to know how people feel.

Quantitative method:

The quantitative method is a research methodology focused on the collection of quantifiable data through surveys, interviews and questionnaires, in order to be able to perform a statistical analysis of all the data collected and thus be able to perform an effective analysis of how many people are affected by the main topic of the research and how it affects them.

Scientific method:

The scientific method is a research method used primarily to acquire scientific knowledge. It is important to use the correct terminology to approach the scientific system in a rigorous and reliable way. It should be based on experience and measurement, following the rules of argumentation, in an ideology closer to reality and the result of a process independent of the researcher's beliefs. On the other hand, it tries to improve the analysis of results by basing its information on evidence and rigorous research adequate to determine how a given question works.

Synthetic analytical method:

This approach involves two inverted mental processes operating simultaneously: analysis and synthesis. Analysis is a logical process that divides things into parts and attributes, into many relationships, properties and components. The analytical method or method of empirical analysis is a model of scientific investigation based on direct experience and empirical logic. It is the most widely used science in both the natural and social sciences. This method analyzes the phenomenon under study, i.e., it breaks it down into its basic elements.

RESULTS

The following results were obtained by conducting several interviews with teaching physicians who are actively involved in the training of medical students:

Table 1.

Interview Questionnaire

Interviewees/ Questions	Teacher N1	Teacher N2	Teacher N3	Teacher N4	Teacher N5
What do you consider to be the fundamental role of the teaching physician in the training of medical students in obstetric emergency care?	The teaching physician plays an essential role in providing guidance and leadership in the training of medical students in obstetric emergency care. Their primary function is to guide students in the	The fundamental role of the teaching physician is to act as a role model, showing students how to apply ethical and humanistic principles in the care of patients in emergency obstetric situations.	In the training of students for obstetric emergency care, the teaching physician plays a crucial role in facilitating active and experiential learning. Their role includes creating	The teaching physician acts as a facilitator of the development of teamwork skills by teaching students to collaborate effectively with other health professionals in the care of obstetric	The teaching physician plays a key role in fostering resilience and stress management skills in medical students, preparing them to face the emotional challenges inherent in emergency obstetric situations.

	development of clinical skills, technical knowledge and clinical judgment necessary to address critical obstetric situations.	In addition to transmitting medical knowledge, he/she fosters values such as compassion, empathy and respect for patients.	simulated environments and promoting hands-on participation, allowing students to apply their theoretical knowledge in realistic situations.	emergencies. This involves promoting clear communication, efficient coordination and shared decision making.	He or she also guides students in developing skills for self-reflection and continuous learning in this demanding clinical context.
What are the main challenges you face in teaching students in this field and how do you address those challenges?	One of the key challenges is the variability in students' clinical experience. To address this, I implement strategies that balance clinical exposure, such as supervised rotations and realistic simulations, to ensure that all students	Time management is a common challenge when teaching obstetric emergencies. To overcome this obstacle, I establish a structured curriculum that prioritizes critical concepts and skills. I also encourage	The diversity of learning styles among students can be a challenge when teaching obstetric emergencies. To address this problem, I implement varied pedagogical approaches, such as	Limited exposure to obstetric emergencies in real clinical settings can be a challenge. To overcome this, I encourage collaboration with medical simulation centers and promote the use of realistic simulations	Constant updating of pedagogical content and practices is a challenge in an evolving medical field. To address this concern, I actively participate in continuing education programs, collaborate with

	acquire essential skills regardless of differences in their prior experience.	efficiency in clinical practice and use technological tools to improve the accessibility of educational resources.	lectures, hands-on activities, and the use of interactive educational technologies, to accommodate different learning styles and enhance understanding.	to provide students with hands-on experiences that mirror obstetric emergency situations in a safe and controlled manner.	experts in the field, and promote educational research to integrate the most recent advances in the training of trainees in obstetric emergencies.
How do you adapt your approach[w] pedagogical approach to ensure that students acquire effective skills in the management of obstetric emergencies?	I tailor my pedagogical approach considering each student's skills and prior knowledge. I provide personalized opportunities for skill development, making sure to address each student's specific areas of improvement in the management	I proactively integrate clinical practice through the use of realistic simulations. This includes obstetric emergency scenarios that allow students to apply their knowledge in a controlled environment,	I implement problem-based learning strategies, where students face specific clinical cases of obstetric emergencies. This fosters critical thinking and problem solving, allowing students to develop effective	I provide constructive feedback on a regular basis to improve students' skills. I use formative and summative assessments to measure their progress and adjust my pedagogical	I incorporate educational technologies as complementary tools for learning. Interactive platforms, virtual simulators and multimedia resources help students visualize and practice

	of obstetric emergencies.	facilitating effective skill acquisition and rapid decision making.	skills for the management of emergency situations.	approach according to individual and collective needs.	procedures, contributing to the acquisition of effective skills in the management of obstetric emergencies.
What strategies do you use to encourage active student participation and promote hands-on learning in emergency obstetric situations?	I design interactive simulation scenarios that mimic obstetric emergency situations. These scenarios allow students to actively participate, make decisions in real time and apply their knowledge in a practical and controlled environment.	I encourage discussions based on real clinical cases to engage students in analysis and problem solving. This strategy promotes active participation by allowing students to apply theoretical concepts to specific clinical situations.	I implement role-plays where students assume specific roles in obstetric emergency situations. This gives them the opportunity to practice communication, decision-making and teamwork skills, encouraging	I facilitate opportunities for hands-on practice in simulated clinical settings, such as virtual delivery rooms or simulation mannequins. These practices allow students to realistically experience procedures and	I encourage collaborative projects where students work in teams to address obstetric emergency cases. This strategy not only promotes active participation, but also enhances teamwork and problem-solving skills in a clinical setting.

			active participation and hands-on learning.	protocols, promoting hands-on, active learning.	
How do you integrate ethics and cultural sensitivity in teaching obstetric emergency care, considering patient diversity?	Design obstetric emergency scenarios that reflect the cultural diversity of the population. This allows students to face situations that consider ethical and cultural aspects, promoting sensitivity and cultural awareness in medical care.	I facilitate discussions and analysis of ethical and cultural cases related to obstetric emergencies. These cases challenge students to consider ethical and cultural factors when making clinical decisions, encouraging reflection and the development of diversity-sensitive skills.	I integrate specific educational sessions on cultural sensitivity in obstetric care. These sessions address topics such as cultural practices related to childbirth, preferences in medical care, and respect for the beliefs and values of different communities.	I collaborate with culturally competent healthcare professionals to provide perspectives and experiences in obstetric emergency care. This allows students to learn from experts who understand the specific ethical and cultural dimensions of different patient groups.	I implement assessments that include cultural competency in the management of obstetric emergencies. This ensures that students are able to apply ethical principles and respect cultural diversity in providing effective and sensitive obstetric care.

What are the educational technologies or methodologies that you find most effective for training students in this specific field?	The use of advanced simulators specific to obstetric emergencies allows students to practice procedures in a controlled environment. These simulators replicate realistic situations, enhancing students' ability to effectively manage obstetric emergencies.	The implementation of virtual and augmented reality technologies offers immersive experiences. This allows students to explore virtual birthing environments, practice procedures and improve their understanding of anatomy, contributing significantly to obstetric emergency training.	The use of interactive online educational platforms facilitates access to up-to-date learning resources. These platforms can include teaching modules, interactive case studies and assessments, providing flexibility for students to learn at their own pace.	The development of educational mobile applications specific to obstetric emergencies provides learners with instant access to relevant information and learning tools. These applications can include instructional videos, interactive clinical cases and protocol reminders.	Creating simulation environments that encourage team practice is essential. This can include simulations in which medical students work together with other healthcare professionals, enhancing the necessary communication and coordination skills.

How do you engage students in hands-on experiences or simulated situations to better prepare them to deal with obstetric emergencies in a real-world setting?	I organize regular sessions of obstetric emergency simulations that replicate realistic scenarios, allowing students to face critical situations and practice decision making under pressure in a controlled environment.	I facilitate clinical rotations in obstetric care settings where students can actively participate in emergency management. This direct hands-on experience gives them the opportunity to apply their theoretical knowledge in real clinical situations.	I promote student participation in interdisciplinary teams dedicated to solving clinical cases of obstetric emergencies. This collaboration fosters the integration of knowledge and skills, preparing students for real clinical situations.	I use high-fidelity simulation mannequins for hands-on training. Students can perform obstetric procedures, such as neonatal resuscitation or performing simulated deliveries, improving their technical skills and confidence in emergency situations.	I encourage student participation in networked simulation programs, where they collaborate with other educational institutions and simulation centers, which broadens exposure to a variety of obstetric emergency scenarios and promotes the exchange of best practices between institutions.

What is your opinion on the importance of continuing education for teaching physicians in the field of obstetric emergency care and how do you ensure you stay current on best practices and medical advances?	I believe that continuing education is crucial in the field of obstetric emergency care because of the constant evolution of medical practices and technologies. Continuous updating ensures that teaching physicians are equipped with the latest knowledge, which translates into more effective teaching.	I value active participation in congresses, symposia and scientific events specialized in obstetrics and gynecology. These meetings provide opportunities to learn about the latest advances, exchange experiences with colleagues and access cutting-edge research in the field.	I establish collaborations with medical professionals specialized in obstetric emergencies. This interaction facilitates the exchange of knowledge and experiences, allowing me to keep abreast of best practices and the latest approaches in the management of critical situations.	I actively engage in continuing education programs, such as specialized courses and workshops in obstetric emergencies. These programs provide a structured framework for learning new techniques, updating protocols and strengthening specific pedagogical skills for student training.	I maintain a close connection with clinical research by participating in the supervision of research projects and clinical studies related to obstetric emergencies. This allows me to incorporate the latest scientific findings into my teaching, ensuring that students are exposed to the most current and relevant information.

Note: Own elaboration

TEACHING PHYSICIAN'S STRATEGY FOR THE DEVELOPMENT OF SKILLS IN OBSTETRIC EMERGENCY CARE IN THE MEDICAL STUDENT

Fundamentals of the strategy for the development of skill in obstetric emergency care in the medical student.

SKILLS AND COMPETENCIES

According to the Ministry of Health (2021), skills and competencies refer to the specific actions performed by the student that involve the application of intellectual abilities together with physical or motor skills, which are directed by methods, systems or procedures. Competencies and aptitudes: competencies refer to intellectual abilities, while aptitudes are related to physical or motor skills in the development process (Díaz Barriga, 2011).

For skills and competencies to be truly effective, they must be employed in accordance with established rules, norms, methods, systems or procedures. By acquiring in-depth knowledge and solid skills in these aspects, superior results will be obtained by putting the corresponding skills and abilities into practice (Secretaría de salud, 2021).

Emergency obstetric complications

Obstetric complications refer to health problems that arise during the gestational period. These problems have the potential to affect the health of the mother, the baby, or both. Some women may have preconception health conditions, which could lead to complications during pregnancy (Office for Women's Health, 2022).

Even among women who were in good health before conceiving, the development of complications during pregnancy can raise the level of risk associated with the maternal condition. Receiving regular prenatal care early in pregnancy can help reduce the likelihood of complications by allowing health care providers to diagnose, treat or manage conditions before they become more serious problems.

Prenatal care can also contribute to the detection of mental health disorders associated with pregnancy, such as anxiety and depression (US Department of Health and Human Services, 2024).

Obstetric complications, by their unforeseen nature, carry a significant risk that requires immediate attention, given their potential to generate lasting sequelae in the long-term health and well-being of the individual. Occurrences known as obstetric emergencies arise from factors that affect both the fetus and the mother, posing a serious threat to her health and life (Oldland et al., 2020). Specialized personnel handle these situations because of the urgency. Staff involvement in these situations expedites decision-making processes and provides hands-on assistance. The role of this team member involves providing experiences, psychological care, and optimal care (World Health Organization, 2016).

According to Campos and Loza (2011), training plays a very important role as part of the set of techniques and tools used for planning and implementing strategies to promote organizational progress in a company. Through training, employees' skills are enhanced to effectively perform their job responsibilities. Since training is a continuous process that aims to improve effectiveness and efficiency in the execution of tasks concomitantly with the improvement of performance, job satisfaction and innovative capacity of workers (Campos and Loza, 2011) (Campos and Loza, 2011).

According to Jimenez Pozo (2023), the importance of timely detection of pathologies in pregnant women is evident in order to prevent possible complications that can be fatal. Therefore, it is imperative to offer training in obstetric emergencies during the management of childbirth, with the purpose of guaranteeing the competence of health personnel. This approach encompasses various elements, such as trained personnel, availability of drugs, adequate equipment and appropriate infrastructure, among other relevant aspects.

Clinical training involves the inclusion of the student in the particular professional environment. At this point the highest level of representation of the interaction between the curriculum and the healthcare environment is reached. The university hospital is the optimal place for this encounter to take place; it offers an ideal environment for this encounter to occur. The tripartite mission encompassing patient care, education and research must not only be conceptualized but also implemented as a tangible reality; rather than merely acknowledging its existence, it must be actively carried out in practice (Millán Núñez, 2008).

In this regard, Millán Núñez (2008) considers it essential that all medical care services be integrated into the educational environment, including hospitalization, consultation rooms, operating rooms, emergency and intensive care areas, technical and examination laboratories, as well as the primary care segment, among others, so that the time students spend in these areas, sometimes accompanied by their mentor or practice instructor (two thirds of the time) or practicing independently (one third of the time), is maximally productive.

Structure of the strategy for the development of obstetric emergency care skills in medical students.

The structure of an effective strategy for the development of skills in obstetric emergency care among medical students should encompass a number of essential components to foster emergency response skills in students requires the implementation of various strategies, some elements of the structure are presented below:

Planning:

It is essential to be prepared by developing an emergency communication plan prior to the eventuality of a critical situation. This plan should contemplate possible accidental scenarios specific to the facility that require the activation of emergency protocols (Supersalud, 2021).

Communication Channels

Identify the means of communication to be used during an emergency situation. According to Ruiz (2024) these channels may include:

- Internal communication: implement a structured internal communication system to ensure that the emergency response team remains adequately informed.

- External Communication: Establish the appropriate means of external communication to keep the authorities, the media and the general public informed.

- Communication with those affected: Interaction with impacted individuals: implement a communication mechanism with those affected by the emergency situation, in order to provide timely information and assistance.

Similarly, Supersalud (2021) indicates that effective communication is of utmost importance in emergency contexts in order to safeguard the safety and integrity of affected individuals. In times of crisis, it is essential to use clear and concise language to convey information effectively and accurately without causing confusion or panic.

Likewise, Supersalud (2021) consider that emergency communication involves the real-time transmission of instructions, warnings and updates, emphasizing the critical importance of each spoken or written word. It is essential to use simple language and refrain from using technical jargon or complex terminology that may be difficult for a general audience to understand.

In addition, Supersalud (2021) indicates that it is advisable to use concise and simple sentences to improve understanding and minimize misinterpretations. It is essential to convey information clearly and precisely, avoiding ambiguities or double meanings that may lead to confusion or misinterpretations. In this regard, the use of bulleted or numbered lists can significantly facilitate the organization and structured presentation of information, thus improving readability. The use of enumerations makes it possible to highlight key aspects and simplify reading, which contributes to the comprehension of information in contexts of pressure or emergency.

Likewise, they consider in Supersalud (2021) that it is crucial to highlight the need to use a tone of voice that is firm but calm when communicating in emergency situations. Instilling a sense of confidence and serenity can be beneficial in mitigating the anxiety of individuals, favoring the creation of a serene and peaceful environment in chaotic situations. Emergency communication requires a clear and precise approach. Adopting a clear and concise communication style, using accessible vocabulary, short and structured sentences, as well as maintaining a calm tone, is crucial during critical situations, facilitating effective message delivery and prompt and appropriate action.

Communication and empathy

The communication process is a fundamental component of the medical art according to (Hafferty, 1994) cited by Maza-de la Torre et al., 2023), which is currently embodied in the skilled contemporary communicator who prioritizes observation and active listening, followed by critical thinking and reflection to articulate information effectively. Communication plays a fundamental role in maintaining the art of medicine through the physician. Moreover, it is a determining factor that patients prioritize when selecting their healthcare provider, as people in poor health often choose physicians based on their communication skills and compassionate demeanor. Unfortunately, this attribute is lacking in most healthcare professionals and is progressively becoming more prevalent.

According to Alcorta-Garza et al. (2005) empathy is recognized as one of the core competencies of medical education in the 21st century, playing a vital role in doctor-user communication. It refers to the competence to understand the experiences and emotions of another individual, whether the patient in question or those close to him or her, together with the skill to transmit this understanding to the affected person. This concept has been theoretically and empirically linked to various attributes, such as respect, pro-social behavior, moral thinking, positive attitudes towards the elderly, clinical skills in obtaining medical histories and physical examination, satisfaction in the physician-patient relationship, quality of the therapeutic relationship and favorable clinical outcomes.

Empathy as stated by Esquerda et al. (2016) encompasses not only emotional aspects, but also involves fundamental components: cognitive, understanding and communication. Numerous studies have established a positive correlation between higher levels of empathy, effective communication and competence in patient-resident management, leading to greater clinical competence.

Specifically, higher levels of empathy are related to greater ease for patients to express their symptoms and concerns, resulting not only in better medical history taking and diagnostic accuracy, but also in greater patient engagement, health education and overall quality of care, leading to reduced stress for the health care provider. Lately, a connection with ethical competence has also been established, increasing the consideration of emotional and relational elements in the analysis and resolution of these types of disputes, as well as the relevance of narrative medicine has been recognized (Spanish Society of Medical Oncology, Women's Breast Cancer Federation, Novartis Oncology, 2008).

Medicine, according to Kraus, (2017), is based on several scientific disciplines and involves the interaction between two human beings: the physician and the patient. Effective communication is at the core of this connection. It is important to recognize that beyond these two individuals lies a broader social context, as the patient is not just a sick individual, but rather a father, a mother, a sibling, a grandparent, who is intricately woven into a larger, more elaborate web. In the curricula of university education, this statement lacks a prominent presence and does not receive due attention, despite its fundamental importance in the training of a medical professional. The deficit present in educational programs needs to be addressed. Mastery of communication skills is essential to ensure optimal quality in patient-provider relationships. Patient satisfaction depends to a large extent on the success of this interaction. Empathy is a crucial element in the patient-physician relationship, but it should not be confused with sympathy. The former implies achieving understanding, tuning in, learning to empathize with others and understanding their emotions, frustrations and fears. Developing competencies in this area involves becoming familiar with the patient's concerns and anxieties, as well as acquiring skills in communication strategies to mitigate and calm such concerns in an effective and practical way (Maza-de la Torre et al., 2023).

Use of standardized procedures and checklists

In the contemporary context of high-risk pregnancy care, the implementation of standardized procedures and checklists is required as an integral part of safety and quality practices. These tools can help ensure that all necessary steps are followed in the management of an obstetric emergency.

- Standardized procedures: Standardization of procedures consists of the implementation of standardized methods and protocols for the execution of various tasks within an entity. Within the field of medical education, standardization has the potential to improve the quality, productivity and efficiency of educational processes (Becciu, 2023).

- Checklists: Checklists serve as valuable tools to ensure completion of all steps within a process or procedure. In the field of medical education, checklists can play a crucial role in assessing learners' performance in specific activities, promoting thorough evaluation that helps to improve efficiency and foster evidence-based decision making (Balderix, 2024).

- Benefits of Standardization and Checklists: These strategies can decrease risks, improve compliance with standards and obligations, make the production chain more efficient, and elevate process clarity4. In addition, they facilitate the training and mentoring of new students, since well-defined procedures facilitate the incorporation of new team members and reduce adaptation time (Obando, 2023).

- Use in Medical Education: Within the medical education setting, standardization of procedures and the use of checklists can be employed for clinical skills instruction, evaluation of student performance, and implementation of protocols for patient care.

Team collaboration training

Team collaboration plays a key role in emergency contexts. A well-coordinated team has the ability to work more efficiently and effectively.

According to Beca et al. (2011) states that the critical need to integrate competencies related to team collaboration has been highlighted as one of the main goals of upcoming medical education. Clinical settings, which vary in size and complexity, accommodate learners from different disciplines and can serve as an exceptional avenue for this type of learning. The aforementioned practice, as long as it involves students delineating their roles and contributions to patients as complementary actions within the concept of experiential learning. Therefore, by allowing student participation in the health care team without compromising the quality of care provided, institutions can meet current accreditation requirements for health care facilities.

According to the findings in the study by Beca et al. (2011), it can be deduced that, although students are not commonly perceived as significant contributors to the work of health personnel, they can play a role that requires greater specificity, which implies the acquisition of corresponding skills. This will enhance the training of future medical professionals, promote effective interdisciplinary collaboration in health care, and improve the quality of patient care. Although this study has qualitative research characteristics that make it difficult to generalize conclusions, it reveals the specific reality of a public hospital, which leads to consider that such reality may be analogous in other health institutions. It is suggested that medical students be integrated as members of the health staff in educational hospital settings, and that the necessary skills to collaborate in interdisciplinary teams be included in the medical training curriculum (Beca et al., 2011).

Simulation in obstetrics

Simulation scenarios offer healthcare professionals the opportunity to exercise and improve their skills in a carefully controlled and safe environment. These scenarios can simulate a variety of obstetric emergency events, providing healthcare professionals with the opportunity to train and improve their response capabilities.

According to Gaba (2004) simulation is presented as a very useful tool in health-related disciplines, due to its ability to accelerate students' acquisition of knowledge and promote their capacity for self-evaluation. Simulation enables the application of trial and error as a form of feedback, thus preparing students for their subsequent experience in real clinical settings. Simulation is a method used to replicate or enhance a real-life experience that is often imbued with naturalistic elements, where the simulated practice substantially mirrors or replicates aspects of the real world in a fully interactive manner.

According to Lopez et al. (2013), its benefits include the following:

1) They significantly enhance learning by complementing traditional teaching methods.

2) They allow the technique to be repeated as many times as required.

3) Students acquire knowledge through the process of making mistakes and subsequently developing new learning.

4) Carefully designed and safe environments are provided, ranging from basic facilities such as a consultation room to conduct an obstetric assessment, to more advanced configurations such as a delivery room unit to provide care for a patient in labor.

5) They facilitate subsequent feedback or analysis in real time, providing students with the opportunity to identify their errors, reflect on them and make corrections to clinical and coordination issues (Lopez et al., 2013).

Clinical simulation in the field of obstetrics according to Altamirano- Droguett, (2019) represents an important contribution to the education and skill development of obstetrical students. The various selected types of low-, medium-, and high-fidelity simulations enhance discovery-based, problem-based, experiential, and meaningful learning. In addition, they exhibit organizational and self-regulatory dimensions to stimuli, based on Burke's and Russell's models, thus manifesting complexity and fidelity very close to reality. Therefore, the environment, senses, language and interpersonal relationships interact with each other, approaching in-hospital clinical contexts. This has improved the safety and confidence of students in the nation's Obstetrics and Child Care programs while participating in real-world clinical practices. However, there is a lack of research demonstrating the advancement of these strategies in the preclinical phase of midwifery practice. Therefore, there is a need to implement clinical simulation training programs designed for nurse-midwife educators to enhance the utilization of this technique in undergraduate and graduate settings. This active learning tool plays a crucial role in the educational process and can also be highlighted for its application in educational research studies. In addition, it would be highly beneficial to all midwifery programs and nursing establish a network as professional centers for clinical simulation training, duly recognized and aligned with the institutional policies of each university. This would support the formal integration of this new teaching methodology into the curriculum, which would require a change in the training culture for future generations (Altamirano-Droguett, 2019).

Full patient simulators

These are life-size mannequins that simulate patients, with anatomical dimensions comparable to those of individuals of various ages, from children to adults (Velasco, 2013). These models are distinguished by their capacity for automation through computer systems, which enable the simulation of physiological and pathological conditions, as well as the generation of crisis scenarios that mimic reality. This category includes obstetric models according to Palés and Gomar (2010). The simulation replicates a complete human body, using software that endows the mannequin with all cardiac, vascular and pulmonary functions.

In this regard Palés and Gomar (2010) indicate that the full patient simulator allows students to interact with the robot, become familiar with the clinical scenario and develop a variety of skills that progress from fundamental to more advanced levels. That is, these types of simulators allow for low-fidelity simulation of basic care procedures (such as posture changes, hygiene routines, transfers, etc.), medium-fidelity simulation to assess a particular clinical sign (such as heart sounds), and high-fidelity simulation in crisis situations, preferably.

These full-body patient simulators are generally placed in realistic settings, such as surgical or emergency care areas, to expose students to a hospital environment that closely resembles real-life scenarios (Altamirano-Droguett, 2019).

Training plan as a strategy

The author Jimenez Pozo (2023) proposes a training plan as a strategy for strengthening staff competencies in obstetric emergencies with the following structure:

- Introduction

- Justification

- Scope: The training plan is applicable to the personnel working in the emergency services of the maternal and child health centers of the networks of the Ica region.

- Training plan objectives:

  o Improve human resource capacities of the micro and health networks of the maternal and child health centers.

  o Contribute to substantially modify negative attitudes during emergency care towards pregnant women during childbirth and puerperium, in addition to perinatal death that affects them, especially among the less favored sectors of the population.

  o Improve interaction among employees and thus increase interest in service quality assurance.

- Objectives

  o General Objectives

    ▪ To develop and/or strengthen the labor competencies of professionals working in FON and FONB facilities, in order to improve the efficacy of the management and benefit processes in the management of pregnant women and thus detect pathologies in time.

- o Specific Objectives

    - Identify the learning needs of the participants, based on the problem of maternal-neonatal health in their local reality and in correspondence with the resolution capacity of the health facility and their professional area.

    - Strengthen and develop capabilities in comprehensive health care, through the improvement of competencies for the management of obstetric emergencies during labor and puerperium.

- Goals: To train 100% of the human resources of the health networks responsible for the sexual and reproductive health strategy and those involved in emergency obstetric care processes.

- Strategies:

  - o The strategies to be employed are.

    - Methodology of exposition - dialogue.

    - Conduct skills and abilities workshops.

    - Knowledge evaluation: Pre and Post test

- Conceptual framework

- Actions to be developed: The actions for the development of the training plan are supported by the agendas that will allow attendees to acquire knowledge to take into account the importance of addressing the main obstetric emergencies to detect pathologies in pregnant women in time and skills for the care of normal childbirth that will improve the quality of care of human resources, for this the following topics are being considered:

- Training topics:

  - o Physiology of pregnancy

- o Hypertensive disorders of pregnancy: Preeclampsia, Eclampsia, Fatty liver and HELLP.

- o Hemorrhage in the first half of pregnancy, second half of pregnancy and puerperium.

- o Hypovolemic shock

- o Principles of CPR

- o Puerperal sepsis.

- o Dystocia: anomalies of presentation, shoulder dystocia and altered progression of labor.

- o Assessment of fetal well-being

- o Assessment for referral to an IPRESS

- o Diseases that can complicate pregnancy: thromboembolic events, diabetes and thyroid disease.

- Resources

- Financing

- Budget

- Schedule

GENERAL ASPECTS OF THE PROCEDURE FOR THE VALIDATION OF THE STRATEGY FOR THE DEVELOPMENT OF OBSTETRIC EMERGENCY CARE SKILLS IN MEDICAL STUDENTS.

The general aspects of validating a strategy to improve competence in obstetric emergency care among medical students generally involve multiple steps and crucial considerations. The following are some general aspects that could be integrated into this procedure:

Strategy definition

The first step according to Fescina et al. (2012) involves clearly outlining the strategy established to improve skills in the management of obstetric emergencies. This would encompass the detailed elaboration of the educational objectives, the pedagogical strategies employed, the resources required and the specific audience, in this case, medical students. Strategy can be conceptualized as a systematic approach used to make decisions within a particular context. It is employed for the purpose of achieving one or more pre-established objectives (Westreicher, 2024).

Literature review

According to Villao Rodríguez et al. (2023), a thorough review of the available literature on obstetric emergency skills training and the training of medical students in obstetric emergencies is essential. This review provides a solid foundation for strategy design and helps to identify best practices and areas for improvement, including guidelines for the care of major obstetric emergencies. First, it is imperative to have a robust theoretical foundation that equips trainees with a thorough understanding of obstetric medical fundamentals and procedures. This is further enhanced by hands-on training, which may include simulations and supervised exercises in authentic clinical settings. In addition, continuous assessment and constructive feedback are essential to ensure understanding and continuous improvement of skills.

In this regard, Jimenez Pozo (2023) highlighted the relevance of using questionnaires and other information gathering techniques to corroborate the effectiveness of pedagogical strategies in this area. It is essential to customize the strategy according to the individual needs of the students and the particular characteristics of the clinical setting, in order to ensure a complete and relevant training. The integration of these components effectively cultivates the readiness of future physicians to competently and safely address obstetric emergencies, a crucial aspect of life-saving medical care.

Strategy design

Detailed strategy design is carried out with careful consideration of specific learning objectives, the most effective instructional methods, and appropriate assessment tools. Detailed strategy formulation is carried out with careful consideration of specified learning objectives, optimal instructional methodologies and appropriate assessment tools. This could involve the development of simulation exercises, hands-on training programs, educational materials and other resources essential to the execution of the strategy.

The practice of strategic design according to Conway (2021) involves helping organizations identify opportunities for people centered innovation and align behind a vision of what to build. It integrates a high level of user experience expertise with a strategic business approach. Professionals specializing in design strategy have the ability to integrate a company's diverse capabilities into the innovation, design and development processes.

Strategic design, according to Yuste (2023) as a design approach, is oriented towards solving complex problems and creating value for all stakeholders in an organizational entity. It needs competencies such as integration, visualization and management, focusing on large-scale challenges in the business and social domains.

Advantages of Strategic Design: Proper implementation of strategic design leads to alignment of objectives, needs, key insights and a shared vision, which promotes cohesion among the entire team and stakeholders. The advantages of strategic design include reduced risk of innovation or change as a result of collaborative processes, more effective communication within and between teams and key stakeholders, and increased resource efficiency by eliminating unnecessary spending on prototypes or hypotheses during the build phase (Yuste, 2023).

Pilot implementation

It is common practice to conduct a pilot phase of the strategy before proceeding with its full-scale deployment. At this stage, a trial of the strategy is conducted with a limited number of students for the purpose of identifying potential challenges, modifying procedures as appropriate, and evaluating the effectiveness of the strategy in relation to the achievement of learning objectives.

According to Mercado-Cruza, et al. (2021) in their study states that some of the strategies implemented focused on maintaining communication with outpatients or hospitalized patients through the use of videoconferencing during consultations and rounds conducted via Videoconferencing; however, these strategies pose the disadvantage of requiring policy modifications within hospital settings regarding the use of electronic devices and records.

In general terms, it was concluded that Virtual Clinical Practices have the potential to favor the strengthening of clinical competencies in medical students. In fact, telesimulation represents a particularly valuable strategy in the current educational landscape due to its ability to circumvent the need for students' physical presence. Furthermore, the use of telecommunications for educational and healthcare purposes has the potential to overcome time constraints, increase accessibility, reduce costs, among other benefits (Mercado-Cruza, et al., 2021).

According to Mercado-Cruza, et al. (2021) virtual simulation constitutes an effective tool in the promotion of clinical skills. The implementation of this strategy faces challenges similar to those observed in any educational innovation.

Evaluation of the strategy:

The evaluation of strategies, as stated by López López (2015), involves analyzing the various elements that impact the effectiveness or ineffectiveness of a business or organizational strategy. It is based on coherence, viability and the capacity to adjust to the modifications and possibilities of the environment.

The following are the elements for the evaluation of strategies according to López López (2015):

Strategy Evaluation Process:

In order to assess a strategy, it is imperative to adhere to the steps outlined below:

- Establish evaluation parameters

- Analyze the strategy

- Evaluate the strategy in light of the established criteria.

- Analyze the strengths and areas of improvement of the strategy.

- To propose possible improvements and refinements to the strategy.

- Carry out the implementation of the required improvements and adjustments.

Evaluation of a strategic framework:

The parameters used to evaluate a business strategy include:

- Coherence: it is important to ensure that there are no contradictions between established goals and policies. The organization must maintain cohesion in its actions.

- Resonance: a capacity to adjust to external environmental conditions and to significant transformations occurring in the environment is required.

- Feasibility: relates to the ability to quantify an organization's financial resources, which is generally the main constraint of a strategic plan.

A detailed analysis of the strategy is conducted in order to assess its effectiveness in promoting the development of obstetric emergency management competencies in medical students. This may involve both quantitative and qualitative data collection through surveys, knowledge assessments, performance observations, and participant feedback.

Analysis of results

The data collected during the evaluation are thoroughly analyzed to determine whether the strategy has achieved the established learning objectives. This involves conducting a comparative analysis of the results before and after the implementation of the strategy, identifying trends and patterns, and drawing conclusions about the overall effectiveness of the strategy (Pineda-Leguízamo et al., 2018).

The analysis of results is an essential component in the optimization process of any strategy or campaign. It facilitates the evaluation of performance and the fulfillment of established goals. In strategies, it is crucial to evaluate performance and make informed decisions. Through exhaustive evaluation, the effectiveness of the strategies implemented is determined and it is verified whether the proposed objectives were achieved. It is a tool that provides crucial information on the effectiveness of strategies and areas that need improvement (Cokomik, 2023).

Results Analysis Procedure

To perform an effective performance analysis, it is imperative:

- Establish research objectives and research questions

- Descriptive and exploratory analysis.

- Analyze the results adequately

- Analyze data completeness and methodological approach

- Clearly and succinctly state the findings.

- Highlight the most significant conclusions.

Reviewing the effectiveness of the business strategy: scrutiny of the effectiveness of the business strategy involves assessing the performance and results achieved through the implementation of the specified strategy. [3]It facilitates the evaluation of the effectiveness of the strategy and the fulfillment of the pre-established objectives.

Check for plagiarism

Report and dissemination of results:

Through a comprehensive report, the complete process of development, implementation and evaluation of the validated strategy is detailed, also presenting the conclusions and recommendations derived from the study. This report can be disseminated to the academic and medical community through scientific publications, conference presentations and other communication channels.

Analysis of the results of skill development strategies

By conducting an analysis of the results of a skills development strategy, according to Kirkpatrick's model, it is elaborated with the objective of evaluating the impact on traditional training programs. His method comprises four levels: response, learning, performance and results. Each element is important and its absence is inconceivable. As the process progresses, it becomes more complex and time consuming, but produces invaluable data (Velázquez, 2024).

The Kirkpatrick model is widely recognized for evaluating training programs by establishing a data-backed chain of evidence that validates the outcomes of the learning process and its implications for organizations, known as Return on Expectations (ROE) (Didactic School, 2024).

Developed a four-level model for evaluating training effectiveness:

- Reaction

- Learning

- Behavior

- Results

According to Miranda (2021) Jack Phillips proposed a six-level model to evaluate the return on investment in training and development:

- Level 1: Reaction

- Level 2: Learning

- Level 3: Application

- Level 4: Impact

- Level 5: Return on investment

- Level 6: Results

Robert O. Brinkerhoff, developed the "Five Levels of Evaluation" model that focuses on:

- Reaction

- Learning

- Application

- Impact

- Return on investment

These authors have made substantial contributions to the field of training evaluation and skills development by offering conceptual frameworks and models that can be customized for the analysis of specific strategies in organizations.

It is essential to adhere to a systematized approach that enables a rigorous evaluation of the impact of the strategy. The following is a general guideline for conducting this analysis:

1. Definition of Objectives

   - Determine the specific objectives to be achieved through the implementation of the skills development strategy.

   - Define clear and quantifiable parameters for each goal.

2. Data Collection

   - Collect relevant information before and after the implementation of the strategy.

   - Employ various techniques such as surveys, interviews, performance evaluations and other methods to gather information of both a quantitative and qualitative nature.

3. Quantitative Analysis

   - Examine the numerical data collected in order to evaluate the quantitative impact of the strategy.

   - Compare previous and subsequent results to determine improvements in specific areas.

4. Qualitative Analysis

   [3]- Analyze elements of a qualitative nature such as participant satisfaction, changes in attitudes or perceptions, and opinions provided in a qualitative manner.

5. Identification of Strengths and Areas of Opportunity

   • Identify the results obtained in relation to the defined objectives.

   • Identify areas where the strategy can be improved or adjusted for future implementation.

6. Performance Impact

   • Examine the effect of the skill development strategy on performance at the individual and organizational level.

   • Examine whether concrete progress has been made in terms of productivity, efficiency or labor quality.

7. Feedback and Future Plans

   - Obtain feedback from participants and stakeholders involved in the process.

   - Use the results of the analysis to refine the strategy and formulate future skills development initiatives.

DISCUSSION OF RESULTS

Through an exhaustive review of the answers provided by the five teaching physicians specialized in obstetric emergencies, a wealth of pedagogical approaches and strategies applied in the training of medical students in this specific field was evidenced. All this taking into account that each teacher offered a unique perspective on the fundamental role of the teaching physician, the challenges inherent in the teaching process, the adaptation of pedagogical approaches, the promotion of active participation, the integration of ethics and cultural sensitivity, the effectiveness of educational technologies, and the preparation of students to face obstetric emergency situations in real contexts.

Regarding the fundamental role of the teaching physician, the importance of guiding and leading in the development of clinical skills, as well as acting as an exemplary role model in both ethical and humanistic principles, is emphasized. In addition, the role of facilitating active and experiential learning, fostering teamwork, and cultivating resilience and stress management skills among students is emphasized.

Challenges faced by faculty in this area include variability in the clinical experience of students, effective time management, diversity of learning styles, limited exposure to obstetric emergencies in real clinical settings, and the need to constantly stay current in the face of an ever-evolving medical field.

Regarding the adaptation of the pedagogical approach, the need to individualize learning to address the different skills and prior knowledge of students is emphasized. The importance of integrating realistic simulations, using problem-based learning strategies, offering constructive feedback on a regular basis and making use of educational technologies is also emphasized.

Strategies to encourage active student participation range from interactive scenario design to case-based discussions, role-playing, practice in simulated environments, and collaborative projects. Each of these strategies is intended to promote hands-on, participatory learning. Within the realm of ethics and cultural sensitivity, teachers stress the importance of designing scenarios and cases that reflect the cultural diversity of the population.

Finally, it should be noted that the importance of continuing education for teaching physicians is unanimously recognized, highlighting active participation in scientific events, collaboration with specialized professionals, adherence to continuing education programs, supervision of research and clinical studies as fundamental strategies for keeping up to date and providing relevant and effective teaching.

CONCLUSIONS

In retrospect, when examining the responses of the teaching physicians specialized in obstetric emergencies, the convergence in the importance assigned to the fundamental role they play in the training of medical students stands out. They all agree that acting as guides, leaders and role models is essential for the development of clinical skills, clinical judgment and ethical principles in future health professionals.

As these faculty shared their experiences, a number of common challenges faced in teaching obstetric emergencies emerged. Variability in student clinical experience, time management, diversity of learning styles, and limited exposure to real cases emerged as significant obstacles. However, each faculty member addressed these challenges with specific strategies, highlighting the need for flexibility and adaptability in their pedagogical approach.

At the pedagogical level, adaptation became a common thread, with teachers emphasizing the importance of adapting their teaching methods to the individual needs of students, integrating realistic simulations, problem-based learning and educational technologies, such a personalized approach proving essential to ensure that each student acquired effective skills in the management of obstetric emergencies.

Finally, the need for continuing education for teaching physicians in the field of obstetric emergency care was highlighted as a unified conclusion. Participation in scientific events, collaboration with experts, continuing education programs, and supervision of clinical research were identified as key strategies to stay current and thus provide informed and relevant teaching.

BIBLIOGRAPHY .

1 . Sanchez. Perception nante la simulación clínica obstétrica en estudiantes de medicina humana de una Universidad Privada de Lima - Perú 2021. [Online]; 2021 [cited 2024 January 31]. Available from: https://hdl.handle.net/20.500.14308/3315.

2 . Campoverde A&. From the memories of knowledge transmission to the foundations of pedagogical mediation. [Online].; 2021 [cited 2024 January 31]. Available from: http://dspace.uazuay .edu.ec/handle/datos/11372.

3 . Paredes. Level of knowledge in obstetric emergencies in high-risk pregnant women in obstetrics interns at the Hospital Materno Infantil Carlos Showing Ferrari, 2018. [Online].; 2021 [cited 2024 January 31]. Available from:

http://repositorio.udh.edu.pe/123456789/3010.

4 . Jimenez. Plan de capacitación para el fortalecimiento de competencias del profesional obstetra en emergencias obstetricas de unos centros Materno Infantil, Ica 2023. [Online]; 2023 [cited 2024 January 31]. Available from: https://hdl.handle.net/20.500.12692/130660.

5 . Moreno. Simulated practice in Obstetric Emergencies as a Learning Scenario. [Online]; 2021 [cited 2024 January 31]. Available from:

http://repository.unipiloto.edu.co/handle/20.500.12277/10815.

6 . Gomar F&. Design of a clinical simulation scenario template. A proposal for training in Obstetrics and Midwifery. [Online].; 2024 [cited 2024 January 31]. Available from: https://dx.doi.org/10.33588/fem.2605.1301.

7 . Llano M&L. Professional skills of Internal Medicine specialists to care for pregnant women with associated pathologies. [Online].; 2023 [cited 2024 January 31], Available from: http://scielo.sld.cu/scielo.php?pid=S1815-76962023000300018&script=sci_arttext.

8 . Alcorta-Garza, A., González-Guerrero, J., Tavitas-Herrera, S., & Rodríguez-Lara, F. (2005). Validation of Jefferson's medical empathy scale in Mexican medical students. *Salud mental, 28*(5), 57-63.

9 . Altamirano-Droguett, J. (2019). Clinical simulation: A contribution to teaching and learning in obstetrics. *Educare Electronic Journal, 23*(2), 167-187.

https://doi.org/10.15359/ree.23-2.9

10 Ausubel, D. (1968). *Educational Psychology: A Cognitive View.* Holt, Rinehart and Winston.

11 Balderix (2024). *Balderix Academy.* Probability and Statistics: https://www.probabilidadyestadistica.net/checklist-lista-de- verificacion/

12 Beca, J. P., Gomez, M. I., Browne, F., & Browne, J. (2011). Medical students as part of the health care team. *Revista médica de Chile, 139*(4), 462-466. https://doi.org/10.4067/S0034- 98872011000400007

13 Becciu, S. (2023). *fullaudits.com.* What is process standardization, how to apply it and examples:

https://fullaudits.com/estandarizacion-de-procesos-aplicarla-y- examples/

14 Bronfenbrenner, U. (1979). *The Ecology of Human Development: Experiments by Nature and Design.* Harvard University Press.

15 Bruner, J. (1966). *Toward Theory of Instruction.* Harvard University Press.

Cambero Martínez, Y., Santisteban Alba, S., Álvarez Sintes, A., Rodríguez, R., Olazabal, J., and Enamorado, A. (2022). Design of the subject Obstetrics and Gynecology based on competency-based training. *Educación Médica Superior, 36* (3), 1-17.

http://scielo.sld.cu/pdf/ems/v36n3/l561-2902-ems-36-03-e3494.pdf

17 Campos, S., and Loza, P. (2011). *Incidence of the administrative management of the municipal library "Pedro Moncayo" of the city of barra in improving the quality of services and attention to users in 2011. Alternative proposal.* Bachelor's thesis, Universidad Técnica del Norte, Ecuador.

http://repositorio.utn.edu.ec/handle/123456789/1945

18 .Cokomik. (2023). https://conomik.com. Practical guide: how to do an analysis of results: https://conomik.com/como-hacer-un-analisis- de-results/

19 .Conway, A. (2021). *discover.egafutura.com.* what-is-strategy-dissertation-and-why-is-it-important: https://discover.egafutura.com/que-es-el-diseno-de-estrategia-y-por- what-is-it-important/

20 Cunningham, F., Leveno, K., Bloom, S., Dashe, J., and Hoffman, B. (2018). *Williams obstetrics.* McGraw-Hill Education.

21 Díaz Barriga, S. (2011). *El enfoque de competencias en educación; la enseñanza situada.* Mexico City: Perfiles educativos.

22 .didactic school. (2024). https://www.escueladidactica.com/. What is the Kirkpatrick model: https://www.escueladidactica.com/que-es-el- modelo-kirkpatrick/

23 Esquerda, M., Yuguero, O., Viñas, J., and Pifarré, J. (2016). Medical empathy, born or made? Evolution of empathy in medical students. *Atención Primaria, 48* (1), 8-14.

https://doi.org/10.1016zj.aprim.2014.12.012

24 . Fescma, R., De Mucio, B., Ortiz, E., & Jarquin, D. (2012). *Guidelines for the care of major obstetric emergencies.* Pan American Health Organization.

https://www3.paho.org/clap/dmdocuments/CLAP1594.pdf

25 Gaba, D. (2004). The future vision of simulation in health care. *Qual Saf Health Care, 13* (1), 2-10.

https://doi.org/10.1136/qhc.13.suppl_1.i2

26 García, C. (2020). *Knowledge, attitudes and practices on the management of obstetric hemorrhage - red key - MSP in postgraduate students of Gynecology and Obstetrics at the Catholic University of Ecuador, Quito.* Specialist Work, Pontificia Universidad Católica del Ecuador, Quito. http://repositorio.puce.edu.ec/handle/22000/18340?show=full

27 Gardner, H. (1983). *Frames of Mind: The Theory of Multiple Intelligences.* Basic Books.

28 Ginoris Quesada, O., Addine Fernández, F., and Turcaz Millán, J. (2006). *Didáctica General.* LATIN AMERICAN AND CARIBBEAN PEDAGOGICAL INSTITUTE.

29 Greif, D., Bottaro, S., Gómez, F., Grenno, A., Nozar, F., Fiol, V., and Briozzo, L. (2015). Training of gynecology residents in obstetric emergencies using clinical simulation. *Rev Méd Urug, 31* (1), 46-52.

30 Jimenez Pozo, E. (2023). *Plan de capacitación para el fortalecimiento de competencias del profesional obstetra en emergencias obstetricas de unos centros Materno Infantil, Ica 2023.* Master's Thesis, Universidad César Vallejo, Lima.

31 Kolb, D. (1984). *Experiential Learning: Experience as the Source of Learning and Development.* Prentice Hall.

32 Kraus, A. (2017). *Empathy: Notes without repose.* Nexos: https://www.nexos.com.mx/7pA30800

33 López López, V. (2015). *Evaluation of strategies.* Emprendices: https://www.emprendices.co/evaluacion-de-estrategias/

34 Lopez, M., Lopez, S., Ramos, L., & Pato, O. (2013). Clinical simulation as a learning tool. *ma. Cirugia mayor ambulatoria, 18* (1), 27-31.

http://www.asecma.org/Documentos/Articulos/05_18_1_FC_Lo%C2%A6%C3%BCpez.pdf

35 Ludeña , D. (2018). *Simulation in the acquisition of clinical competencies for the management of obstetric emergencies, shoulder dystocia in medical students of the Universidad Técnica Particular de Loja, period September 2013-February 2014.* Medical degree thesis, Universidad Técnica Particular de Loja, Loja.

36 Machado Linde, F., Prieto-Sánchez, M., Sánchez-Ferrer, M., and Nieto, A. (2014). Optimization of clinical practices in the learning of Gynecology and Obstetrics by the medical student. *II International Congress of Teaching Innovation.* Murcia.

37 Maslow, A. (1970). *Motivation and Personality.* Harper & Row.

38 Maza-de la Torre, G., Motta-Ramírez, G., Motta-Ramírez, G., and Jarquin-Hernández, P. (2023). Empathy, effective communication, and assertiveness in current medical practice. *Revista de sanidad militar, 77*(1). https://doi.org/10.56443/rsm.v77i1.371. https://doi.org/10.56443/rsm.v77i1.371.

39 Mercado-Cruza, E., Morales-Acevedo, J., Lugo-Reyes, G., Quintos-Romero, A., and Esperón-Hernández, R. (2021). Telesimulation: a strategy to develop clinical skills in medical students. *Research in Medical Education,* *10*(40), 19-28. https://doi.org/10.22201/fm.20075057e.2021.40.21355. https://doi.org/10.22201/fm.20075057e.2021.40.21355

40 Millán Núñez, J. (2008). The teaching of clinical skills. *Educación Médica,* *11* (1), 21-27.

http://scielo.isciii.es/scielo.php?script=sci_arttext&pid=S1575-18132008000500005&lng=es&tlng=es

41 Miranda, A. (2021). *The 3 best methods for evaluating training effectiveness.* https://es.linkedin.com/pulse/los-3-mejores- methods-for-evaluating-the-effectiveness-of-miranda-rojas.

42 Obando, R. (2023). *What is process standardization, how to apply it.* https://blog.hubspot.es:

https://blog.hubspot.es/sales/estandarizacion-de-procesos

43 .office for women's health. (2022). https://espanol.womenshealth.gov/: https://espanol.womenshealth.gov/pregnancy/youre-pregnant-now-what/pregnancy-complications.

44 Oldland, E., Botti, M., Hutchinson, A., & Redley, B. (2020). A framework of nurses'responsibilities for quality healthcare - Exploration of content validity. *Collegian,* *27*(2), 150-163. https://doi.org/10.1016zj.colegn.2019.07.007

45 World Health Organization. (2016). *Global strategic directions for strengthening nursing and midwifery 2016-2020.* https://www.who.int/publications-detail-redirect/9789240033863

46 Palés, J., and Gomar, C. (2010). The use of simulations in medical education. Teoría de la educación. *Education and culture in the information society, 11* (2), 147-169.

http://www.ub.edu/medicina_unitateducaciomedica/documentos/Lus%20de%20les%20simulacions%20en%20educacio%20medica.pdf

47 Piaget, J. (1976). *The birth of intelligence in the child.* Fondo de Cultura Económica.

48 Pineda-Leguízamo, R., Miranda-Novales, G., & Villasís-Keever, M. (2018). The importance of clinical case reports in research. *Revista alergia México, 65*(1), 92-98.

https://doi.org/https://doi.org/10.29262/ram.v65i1.348

49 Ruiz, E. (2024). https://plandemergencia.com/.

https://plandemergencia.com/comunicacion-en-situaciones-de-crisis/what-are-the-best-strategies-for-communicating-in-emergency-situations-clearly-and-precisely/

50. secretary of health. (2021). *Manual de habilidades didácticas para la formación de instructores de primeros respondientes.* Mexico: Technical Secretariat of the National Council for Accident Prevention.

https://www.gob.mx/cms/uploads/attachment/file/783775/Manual_Formaci_n_Instructors_030321.pdf

51 Skinner, B. (1954). The Science of Learning andthe Art of Teaching. *HarvardEducationalReview, 24*(2), 86-97.

52 Spanish Society of Medical Oncology, Breast Cancer Women Federation, Novartis Oncology (2008). *Empathy, essential in doctor-patient communication.* Spanish Society of Medical Oncology:

https://www.seom.org/seomcms/images/stories/recursos/salaprensa/n
otasprensa/2008/np_guia_empatia.pdf

53 Soler Martínez, C. (2004). Reflections on the term competencies in teaching activity. *EducMedSuper., 18*(1).

54. Supersalud. (2021). *Emergency prevention, preparedness and response plan.* Minsalud, Superintendencia Nacional de Salud. https://docs.supersalud.gov.co/PortalWeb/planeacion/Planes/SST%2 0-%20PlanPPR%20Emergencias2021.pdf.

55 Tapia Villanueva, R., Núñez Tapia, R., Syr Salas, R., and Rodríguez-Orozco, A. (2007). The undergraduate medical internship and clinical competencies. *Educación Médica Superior,, 21* (4). http://scielo.sld.cu/scielo.php?script=sci_arttext&pid=S0864-21412007000400005

56 . Universidad del Azuay. (2023). http://www.uazuay.edu.ec.

https://www.uazuay.edu.ec/estudios-de-grado/carreras/medicina:
https://www.uazuay.edu.ec/estudios-de-grado/carreras/medicina

57 Urra, E., Sandoval, S., & Irribarren, F. (2017). The challenge and future of simulation as a teaching strategy in nursing. *Revista Investigación en Educación Médica, 6(22)*, 119-125.

http://www.scielo.org.mx/scielo.php?pid=S2007-50572017000200009&script=sci_arttext

58 US Department of Health and Human Services. (2024). www.nichd.nih.gov.

www.nichd.nih.gov/health/topics/pregnancy/conditioninfo/complicat ions:

https://www.nichd.nih.gov/health/topics/pregnancy/conditioninfo/co mplications

59 Vázquez Gómez, L., Rodríguez Calvo, M., Arriola Mesa, Y., and Rodríguez Casas, E. (2015). Assessment of clinical skills in third-year medical students. *Edumecentro, 7*(3), 1-12.

60 Velasco, A. (2013). *Clinical simulation and nursing, creating a simulation environment.* Degree work, University of Cantabria. https://metodoinvestigacion.files.wordpress.com/2014/11/simulacic3 b3n-cc3b1inica-y-efermerc3ada-creando-un-ambiente-de- simulacic3b3n-u-de-cantabria.pdf.

61 Velázquez, A. (2024). *QuestionPro*. What is the Kirkpatrick evaluation model: https://www.questionpro.com/blog/es/modelo-de-.

evaluation-kirkpatrick/

62 Villao Rodríguez, L., Yaguana Torres, J., and Lara Arriaga, S. (2023). Strategy for the Development of Skills in Obstetric Emergency Care in the Medical Student. *Ciencia latina.* https://ciencialatina.org/index.php/cienciala/article/download/836l/l 2568?inline=1

63 Vygotsky, L. (1978). *Mind in Society: The Development of Higher Psychological Processes.* Harvard University Press.

64 .westreicher, G. (2024). *what is a strategy?* economipedia: https://economipedia.com/definiciones/estrategia.html

65 World Health Organization (2016). *Managing complications in pregnancy and childbirth: a guide for midwives and doctors.* World Health Organization.

66 .Yuste, G. (2023). https://keepcoding.io/blog. que-es-el-diseno-estrategico/: https://keepcoding.io/blog/que-es-el-diseno-estrategico/

CONTENTS

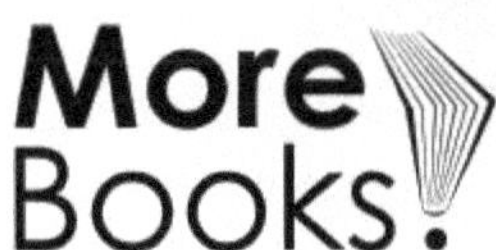

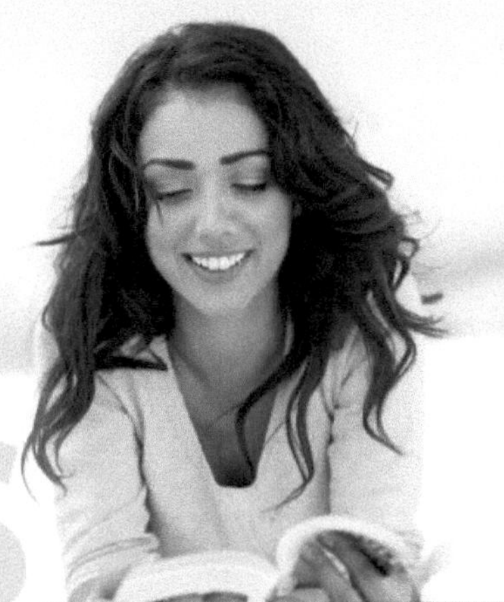

yes
I want morebooks!

Buy your books fast and straightforward online - at one of world's fastest growing online book stores! Environmentally sound due to Print-on-Demand technologies.

Buy your books online at
www.morebooks.shop

Kaufen Sie Ihre Bücher schnell und unkompliziert online – auf einer der am schnellsten wachsenden Buchhandelsplattformen weltweit! Dank Print-On-Demand umwelt- und ressourcenschonend produzi ert.

Bücher schneller online kaufen
www.morebooks.shop

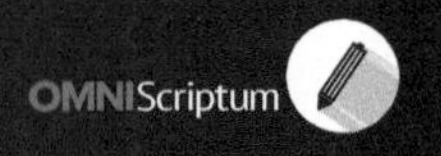

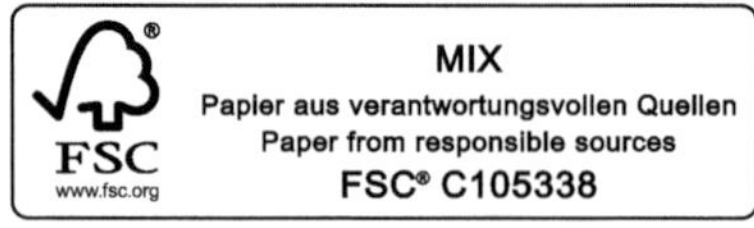

Printed by Books on Demand GmbH, Norderstedt / Germany